PARASITES IN DELUSIONAL PARASITOSIS

An increasing Pandemic of Morgellon's Syndrome

AUTHOR:

Neelam Taneja-Uppal, M.D.

1

ABOUT THE AUTHOR:

Dr. Neelam Uppal, has had many years of experience in Infectious Diseases and internal

Medicine. Dr. Uppal graduated from Christian Medical College in India. From there she

went to New York where she did her internship and then did her Residency in New

Jersey in Internal Medicine. She then did her fellowship in Infectious Diseases in New

York hospital of Queens and Memorial Sloan- Kettering medical Center.

Dr. Uppal is board certified in Infectious Diseases, on the Advisory Board of National

Morgellon's Foundation, Winner of American College of physicians award in 1990, was

quoted in new York Times and several National Television Shows., recently on Rachel

ray show on July 23,2010.

AWARDS AND HONORS:

- PHYSICIAN OF THE YEAR –2006 BY NRCC
-
- MADISON'S WHO'WHO
-
- STANFORD WHO'S WHO
-
- AMERICAN COLLEGE OF PHYSICIANS RESEARCH AWARD-FIRST PLACE-1990

MEMEBERSHIPS:

<u>**AMERICAN COLLEGE OF PHYSICIANS**</u>

INFECTIOUS DISEASE SOCEITY OF AMERICA

FLORIDA INFECTIOUS DISEASE SOCEITY OF AMERICA

AMERICAN MEDICAL ASSOCIATION

FLORIDA MEDICAL ASSOCIATION

PINELLAS COUNTY MEDICAL SOCEITY

FLORIDA ASSOCIATION OF PHYSICIANS
FROM INDIA

AMERICAN ASSOCIATION OF
PHYSICIANS FROM INDIA

PINNELLAS PARK CHAMBER OF
COMMERCE

OVERVIEW

The book is based on my practice of Infectious diseases and discovery of a new parasitic

disease referred to as Morgellon's Disease. My experience made me realize the dilemmas

of the recognition of the disease in the medical community and social implication. It

made me understand how it may be spreading in United States and how it may be

prevented as a Public Health issue. Hence to bring this awareness to the public and

healthcare providers I was compelled to write this book.

A 40 years old woman comes to my office with sores all over body. Complains of

crawling sensations and itching. States she sees threads coming out of her body. She

grabs the hand sanitizer and rubs on her belly and tries to bring out stuff. She has been

diagnosed with 'delusional parasitosis'. But in talking to her she is an extremely

intelligent woman. So I decide to investigate and what I have discovered is in this book.

TABLE OF CONTENTS

CHAPTER I

What led me to write this book is that I can educate the people with the disease, their families and caretakers that have to deal with these patients and the health care professionals that are looking for some answers unraveled a mysterious Disease, that has baffled the smartest of physicians. See how the pets can transmit parasites which may not be identified by your healthcare provider, and you could be deemed 'DELUSIONAL' A woman in her forties comes to my office with sores and itching and feeling crawling sensations on her skin. The husband is ready to divorce her because she keeps acting 'Crazy' trying to show him bugs coming out of her. But he sees nothing. The patient is deemed 'Delusional'. But I realized what the patient was feeling due to her parasitic involvement and calmed the husband. The patient is now feeling better.

CHAPTER II

EPIDEMIOLOGY

Most patients that were seen were coming from California,

Texas and Florida. The common things in these places are the weather, which is tropical. It is hot and all these states are on the water

IMMIGRATION:

Parasites are prevalent in the tropical climate third world countries. With a lot people migrating from these countries, the parasites came with them. May be their pets got infested. The pets go outside and sometimes even eat off the road another dogs' feces. A lot of people clean the litter of the cats.

TRANSMISSION:

On retrospective analysis it was fund that ball patients had one thing in common that is, pets. And the pet was either sick or had worms that were treated.

The review of the life cycles of most of the parasites in the pets shows that the pets ate the intermediate host of most of the parasites.

The hot weather supports the optimum temperature for the proliferation of these organisms.

Also the availability of the water helps in the transmission of the larval stage.

For example, if the dogs had worms, he did his thing and cleaned himself, but the eggs could have stayed on. And then the owner slept with the dog, had the dog on his lap or played with the dog the eggs can get attached to the hand, get embedded in the nails and then subsequently get injected.

The water in these areas helps transmission of the larval forms. People take dogs on some of the beaches. The larval forms can get hatched and swim around and then penetrates the skin of a human being and they get the parasite.

Also the fleabites can transmit the eggs and then either deposits it in their bite or feces.

Evidence based Medicine:

The standard of practice for the diagnosis of parasites is to send stool ova and parasites under microscope.

But the regular commercial Lab Personnel is not trained. So even if you send a clearly positive specimen, the result comes back negative

When the doctor looks at the result and tells the patient that their test is negative; they do not have parasites.

And thus' the patient is labeled 'CRAZY'

CHAPTER III

Parasites from Pets:

There are a lot of parasites that can be transmitted by the cats and dogs.

These can be:

Hookworm

Tapeworm

Toxoplasma

Toxocara canis and Catis

Cat Scratch Disease

Dog Heart Worm is Dirofilaria

Fish tapeworm- Ecchinococcus needs dogs or cats as

intermediate host.

Also called Dog tapeworm

Pinworm

Roundworm

Cysticercosis, Tenia soliumm and Tenia saginatta.

The lab results come back borderline positive. So these

organisms could be related to these worms.

CHAPTER IV

NOMENCLATURE:

Morgellon's is referred to as Delusional Parasitosis. It needs to be corrected to unspecified Parasitosis. CDC terms it as 'Unspecified Parasitosis'

WHAT IS UNSPECIFIED PARASITOSIS:

It is a syndrome in which patients present with multiple signs and symptoms. All patients may not have exactly the same symptoms and signs.

SYMPTOMS OF UNSPECIFIED PARASITOSIS

- Rash

- Skin Lesions

- Papules Abscesses

- Ulcers

- Vesicles

- Organisms

- Thread like granules

- Itching

- Fatigue

- Fever

- Chills

- Depression

- Delusions

- Irritability

CHAPTER V

DELUSIONAL PARASITOSIS:

- Delusions (seen patients, because the disease is not recognize and a lot of times patients feel the crawling, seen organisms coming out might be microscopic however the doctor's doesn't see it)** Some of the patients pull threads from a sock and when they visit the doctor they would say that it came out from their skin or on the other parts of their body. And, also because of the stress their experiencing they want the doctor to believe in them.

- Irritability – patients are irritable and anxious because they're trying to convince something to the doctor who doesn't know a thing.

The other persons who also don't know are the commercial laboratories. When I was a medical student there was a professor who used to say, " If the mind doesn't know, the eyes don't see." In this case how many lab technicians in the commercial laboratories that look at the stool specimen and knows how to identify that eggs.

It is very odd and hard to identify an egg; an untrained eye will not see it. When the result comes back it's negative. Sometimes the doctor would tell the patient that it's all in their head but no, it's more in the doctor's head who doesn't know.

I believed that why we have a lot of mis-cases happen because I don't think that the commercial laboratories were equipped enough with a trained personnel to make the diagnosis.

SYMPTOMS OF DELUSIONAL PARASITOSIS

- Rash
- Skin Lesions
- Papules Abscesses

- Ulcers

- Vesicles

- Organisms

- Thread like granules

- Itching

- Fatigue

- Fever

- Chills

- Depression

- Delusions

- Irritability

OTHER SIGNS:

- Weight Loss – significant weight loss

- Multiple Skin Lesions – in different stages

- Anxiety

- Swelling

- Red Areas – due to cellulitis

- Cellulitis

CHAPTER VI

DIAGNOSTIC TESTS:

The other personnel who also don't know are the commercial

laboratories. When I was a medical student there was a

professor who used to say, " If the mind doesn't know, the eyes

don't see." In this case how many lab technicians in the

commercial laboratories that look at the stool specimen and knows how to identify that eggs.

It is very odd and hard to identify an egg; an untrained eye will not see it. When the result comes back it's negative. Sometimes the doctor would tell the patient that it's all in their head but no, it's more in the doctor's head who doesn't know.

I believed that why we have a lot of missed cases happen because I don't think that the commercial laboratories were equipped enough with a trained personnel to make the diagnosis.

CHAPTER VII

LABORATORY TEST:

- CBC

- Chemistry

- Lime Test

- Herpes Test – generalized form kind of lesions

- Strongyloides cross reaction to strongyloides some patients have low positive reaction to Schistosoma

- Schistosoma

- Echinococci - echinococcus, is another test that comes out as low positive

- MRSA – (Methicillin-resistant staphylococcus aureus) detailed about the bacteriology that was presented, a lot of the times the lesion would be positive with MRSA and have not responded with any other antibiotic

  Bacterial

  - MRSA

  - E- coli

  - Pseudonomous

  - Proteus

** Were seen in these lesions, in my first opinion it was a super infection because of the skin, and the second opinion that I have that a lot of these people will have a grand negative in which is a bowel flora that is in the lesions.

** These bacteria were coming into the lesions because of the larva migrans from the bowel to the bloodstreams and into the lesions.

- Stool O & P – I sent out samples and when the results comes in, it's always negative
- Urine – patients complains that seeing lesions or stuff coming out of the urine.

  ** I decided to examine one patient vagina because the patient told me that she found stuff on her privates. Once I open her vagina I saw a finger like white stuff crossing in front of me from one mucosa to the other. That the time I started believing that there is this disease that is called "Morgellans Disease".

- ANA

  ** I also send samples to see if there is autoimmune problem and also to look for lupus

- SED rate
- ANCA – is for vasculitis
- Ankylostoma – which is the hook worm
- Filaria

- Dirofilaria

CHAPTER VIII

PROCEDURES:

- Wound Cultures - we sent out wound cultures, which could be super infections or a suggestions where the worms coming from.

- Skin Biopsy

- Examination of parasite under microscope – patients bringing different parasite moving stuff that were sent to the lab for parasitic microscopic examination, which is usually identified as nothing or ignored or it isn't found.

CHAPTER IX

KNOWN PARASITES DIAGNOSIS

** They do get labeled with a known diagnosis, why… because otherwise you don't get paid. Most of the patients have insurances, so you have to justify the lesions and something that is already known and something that is acceptable to the peers.

- Filaria
- Scabies - maybe resistant kind

    ** The patients get lesions with these classics entry and exit. But can parasites do that? Yes, you see a couple of pairs, hyper pigmentation. They get Koebner's phenomena.

- Larva Migrans - most common diagnosis that I would use on a lot of Morgellon's patients because that's an acceptable diagnosis. A lot of symptoms are what the parasites do. It's a stage of parasites where the larva goes throughout the body and finds the destination or even come back to the bowel. Most of the worms will penetrate the bowels, into the bloodstream and some cases into the lungs.

**I have a patient that had an x-ray and the result came out negative, however the patient is coughing and I can hear something from her lungs. I told my patients to bring me the x-ray film, and we could see small specks all over the x-ray. The patient is going through larva migrans with a pulmonary stage where it goes through the lungs.

** These patients will sometimes tell me that they have chills in the night, sweats in the nights, fever it could be a night or a daytime, that's when they generate the larva. That is a pattern done by filaria, and is done in cycle.

• Tape Worm

• Eccinococcus

• Strongyloides

- Schistosoma

- Roundworm

- Ringworm

- Hookworm

- Pinworm

- Toxocara

CHAPTER X

WHY DID I GET IT?

• Exposure - epidemiology, a lot of cases from Florida, Texas, California, states which are next to the water. These parasites act in a filaria form and one of the modes of transmissions is water. These larvae are migrating in the water, you go in the water, it penetrates and you get it. And also in places with warm or tropical climates.

   ** Why now it's happening not 10 years ago? More immigrants are coming from other parts of the world. Especially, third world countries brought parasites with them. Probably these parasites mutated to our environment and are now infecting places with tropical climate and also places that surrounded by water.

• Low Immunity - it could be any chronic illness or anybody in any medication

   ** I will check their immune system and I will find what is wrong with them by a series of test: immoglubin

deficiency, B cell disorder, T cell disorder. Also, chronic
disease likes diabetes, pulmonary diseases, HIV,
Hepatitis. And autoimmune diseases

• Pets - whether it's being transmitted through mites,
  fleas.

   ** I have a patient who had a sick dog who was
licking her, and now she had   lesions all over her face.
Another patient who used to sleep with her dog came
back positive with dirofilaria, which is a dog hart worm.
A lot of time people do not give anti-parasitic medicines
to the dogs and in these warm climates the dogs and cats
carry worms a lot and they have to be routinely treated.

• Travel - if you travel to a third world country where you
  were exposed. Example of the people was the militaries,
  missionaries. If you went to a place and eat something
  bad and got infected.

• Warm Climate

- Close Contacts - I have patient that I was treating that comes with her sister, now the sister got it, comes with her husband and now the husband got it. Close contacts were they're sharing foods, sleeping beds, using the same furniture's, and towels. The risk considering parasites are in different forms there's the egg, the larva and the adult. And, if it's a filariform there are two types, there is the larva form, which is actually infectious, it doesn't stay in the environment for long but on close contacts the larva form is still infectious you can get it. In the egg form it can stay in dirt, water.

- National Origin - if I see patients with different countries. I had a patient who came from Africa, South America and also one patient from Egypt. He apparently came in with a parasite, which is dormant, and these people have positive results. One of the patients from Africa actually has positive result for trichinella, but treating him for trichinella did not take the disease off, so he has this modified parasite that his harboring which is not being cured with any medication that is around.

CHAPTER XI

HOW DID I GET IT?

- Do you have a dog?

- Do you have a cat? - Who were sick and carrying worms

- Did you work in a pet store?

- Did you go out of the country?

- Did you eat something bad?

- Did you wash hand? - If your working in a high risk environment or if your cleaning your pet, and if the pet is infested with parasites there might be eggs in his body and your handling him, you put the eggs under your nails and you ingest them.

- Did you walk bare footed? - It could be in the beach, on the carpet where the dogs or cats has been there, the eggs or larva can penetrate your feet which can cause you the infection.

CHAPTER IX

WHAT CAN I DO ABOUT?

** It's a big blank. But, there's hope because patients do respond to certain regiments of treatments.

ANTI-PARASITICS

- Mebendazole
- Albendazole
- Ivermectin

- Kwell Lotion

- Permethrin

- Malathion

- Mebendazole Ointment

ANTIBIOTICS

- BACTRIM

- CIPRO

- DOXYCYLIN

- ZYVOX

- IV ANTIBIOTICS

** Also some for anti-fungal…aspergillus's, candida,

CHAPTER XIII

** Research that I started doing, which was accepted by American College Physicians for Presentation

DI-ETHYLCARBAMAZINE IN THE TREATMENT OF MORGELLON'S DISEASE

WHAT DO WE NEED?

- More research

- More money to do the research

- I need you help, to help you - any letters of support, or research grants would me appreciated

CHAPTER XIV

QUESTIONS & ANSWERS

1) Is there a proven treatment that works for everyone?

No, every time I think that may have figured it out, the next patient will be entirely different. I get a treatment that some people respond beautifully to it, and then the next people wouldn't respond at all. That's makes it so hard, each individual case is a brand new thing. So far there's hasn't been anything that works for everyone. But we have some patients that are totally cured by certain treatments, but not everyone responds to these treatments.

2) If any placebo controlled studies done with any patients with Morgellon's, if any following classes of medicines: anti-bacterial, anti-fungal, anti-parasitic, anti-depressions and if not, are any such studies plan?

I think we were alluding to because each situation maybe somewhat unique in terms of exposures to illnesses involved, genetically dispositions. Often treatments were individualized.

CHAPTER XV

DILEMMAS OF DIAGNOSIS OF

MPRGELLON'S DISEASE

LABORATORY TEST:

- CBC

- Chemistry

- Lyme Test

- Herpes Test – generalized form kind of lesions

- Strongyloid – cross reaction to strongylitis some patients have low positive reaction to Schistosoma

- Schistosoma

- Echinococci - echinococcus, is another test that comes out as low positive

- MRSA – (Methicillin-resistant staphylococcus aureus) detailed about the bacteriology that was presented, a lot of the times the lesion would be positive with MRSA and have not responded with any other antibiotic

  Bacterial

  - MRSA

  - E- coli

  - Pseudomonas

  - Proteus

** Were seen these lesions, in my first opinion it was a super infection because of the skin, and the second opinion that I have that a lot of these people will have a grand negative which is a bowel flora that is in the lesions.

** These bacteria were coming into the lesions because of the larva migrans from the bowel to the bloodstreams and into the lesions.

- Stool O & P – I sent out samples and when the results comes in its

- Urine

- ANA

- SED rate

- ANCA

- Ankylostoma

- Filaria

- Dirofilaria

DILEMMA OF THE LABORATORY DIAGNOSIS

The laboratories in America do not have technician well-trained in parasitology detection, especially in the commercial laboratories. The fresh stool needs to be examined in 48 hours, but you don't get the results until after a week. Hence, you get a test result that is negative. But the patient has the symptoms and the parasite; thus, the doctor calls the patient 'delusional', as there is no evidence to the patients' symptoms. And the patient does not get treated and one does not know what to treat the patient with. In a society of 'Evidence based Medicine' the doctor is trained to treat the evidence and not the patient. If the test is negative the Insurance company will not pay the doctor for treating the patient or pay for the medicines

CHAPTER XVI

Persistence of Infection:

Some patients will keep coming back with new lesions. The question then arises that is it a new lesion due to relapse, resistence or re-infection. It could be either one but a lot of times I believe it is re-infection. As the pet may be still infected or carrying the infection . or the pet may be re- infecting the household, the beds the couch, sofa etc. and the patient keeps getting re-infected. Or the pet is just continuing to shed egss. And the eggs can stay potent for a long time. Even on surfaces and beds and chairs leading to re-infections.

Concomitant bacterial Infections:

On several occasions there is concomitant bacterial Infections on th skin lesions,

These could be the skin flora of Staphylococcus epidermidis or aureus or MRSA. Or it could be an enteric pathogen that migrated with the larva of the parasite during the Larva Migrans phase. These are very commonly proteus sp.. They can also be enterococcus, pseudomonas, E.coli etc.

CHAPTER XVII

THE FIBERS:

SITES OF SKIN LESIONS: The lesions very commonly occur initially at the site of the infection. Then the reside in the flexural areas of the body and keep recurring either as the residual infection or re- infection.

THE FIBER COLORS:

Patients see blue fibres which is known to be the shaft of the parasite in the venous phase. The look red in the arterial phase. The white fuzz that comes out is the excreta of the filamentous worms. The sand that comes out is the eggs of the worms. The patients feel it as nodules. Once they itch on it or expel the egg, it becomes an open micro sore evidencing the fact that it is a solid granule that comes out and not the pus as in acne.

The patients very commonly have a concomitant infection with disseminated Herpes Simplex, which is then superinfected with very commonly, MRSA or Proteus.

Most of these patients may also have immune – dysfunction or some other immune compromising disease states.

NEELAM T. UPPAL, M.D.
5840 PARK BLVD.
PINELLAS PARK, FL.-33781
PH.-(727)-547-5232
FAX-(727)-547-5233

1990 – Present: PRIVATE PRACTICE

TRAINING HISTORY:

1988-1990: PGY4&5:FELLOWSHIP:
INFECTIOUS DISEASE
New York Hospital of Queens,
Main street,
Flushing, New York

1985-1987: PGY2&3:RESIDENCY:
INTERNAL MEDICINE

Jersey city Medical Center, 50 Baldwin Ave.,

Jercey City, NJ

1984-1985: PGY1: INTERNSHIP:
INTERNAL MEDICINE

Methodist Hospital, 601, 5th Ave Brooklyn, NY

1978-1984: MEDICAL SCHOOL:
Bachelor of Medicine

&Bachelor of Surgery

Christian Medical College, India

QUALIFICATIONS:

**ABIM : BOARD CERTIFICATION -
2:**Infectious Disease: 1996-2006

ABIM: BOARD CERTIFICATION-1 :
Internal medicine: 1990-2000

ECFMG :1984

M.B.B.S. :1984

AWARDS AND HONORS:

- PHYSICIAN OF THE YEAR –2006 BY NRCC
-
- MADISON'S WHO'WHO
-
- STANFORD WHO'S WHO
-
- AMERICAN COLLEGE OF PHYSICIANS RESEARCH AWARD-FIRST PLACE-1990

MEMEBERSHIPS:

AMERICAN COLLEGE OF PHYSICIANS

INFECTIOUS DISEASE SOCEITY OF AMERICA

FLORIDA INFECTIOUS DISEASE SOCEITY OF AMERICA

AMERICAN MEDICAL ASSOCIATION

FLORIDA MEDICAL ASSOCIATION

PINELLAS COUNTY MEDICAL SOCEITY

FLORIDA ASSOCIATION OF PHYSICIANS
FROM INDIA

AMERICAN ASSOCIATION OF
PHYSICIANS FROM INDIA

PINNELLAS PARK CHAMBER OF
COMMERCE

www.ingramcontent.com/pod-product-compliance
Lightning Source LLC
Chambersburg PA
CBHW071242220526
45468CB00002B/967